All About
COPING with CONFUSION:
DELERIUM and DEMENTIA

By Laura Flynn R.N., B.N., M.B.A., in consultation with her nurse educator associates and physicians who assisted in contributing and editing.

ISBN No: 978 1 896616 59 9

© 2011, 2017 Mediscript Communications Inc.

The publisher, Mediscript Communications Inc., acknowledges the financial support of the Government of Canada through the Canadian Book Fund for our publishing activities.

Printed in Canada

www.mediscript.net

Book and Front Cover design by:
Brian Adamson, www.AdamsonGraphics.net

CF1002010

ALL ABOUT BOOKS
Trusted • Reliable • Certified

- 40+ titles available
- Comply with accreditation and regulatory bodies
- Suitable for caregivers, boomers with elderly parents, health workers, auxiliary health staff & patients
- Self study style with "test yourself" section
- Health On the Net (HON) certified

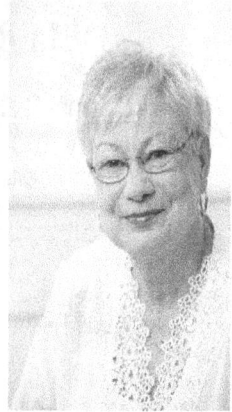

Some of our titles:

Alzheimer's Disease	Arthritis	Multiple Sclerosis
Pain	Strokes	Elder Abuse
Falls Prevention	Incontinence	Nutrition & Aging
Personal Care	Positioning	Confusion
Transferring people	Care of the Back	Skin Care

For complete list of titles go to www.mediscript.net

Contact: 1 800 773 5088
Fax 1800 639 3186 • Email: mediscript30@yahoo.ca

CONTENTS

INTRODUCTION

This book provides basic, non controversial and trusted information that can help a wide spectrum of readers.

The primary objective of the information is to help a person provide effective quality care to a loved one or someone in his or her care.

After reading this material you will have greater confidence in your caregiving role and will know what to do to help the confused person. Equally important, you will better understand the many aspects of confusion in older people.

All the information is reliable and was written by a group of eminent nurse educators who ensured the information complies with best practice guidelines and satisfies the various accreditation and regulatory bodies. Because there is so much unreliable information on the internet, you can be assured the "All About" publications are HON (Health On the Net) certified.

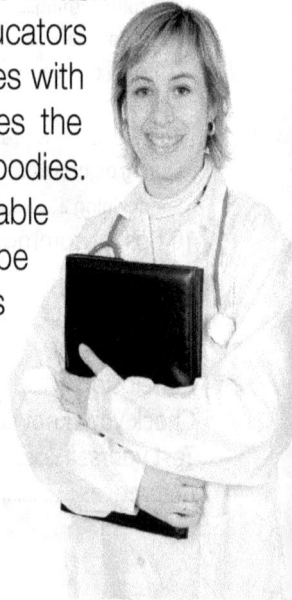

This book can be an invaluable aid to:

- A caregiver caring for a relative or friend;
- A health worker seeking a reference aid;
- Any person involved in health care wishing to expand his or her knowledge.

SOMETHING TO THINK ABOUT...

Wisdom is to see the miraculous
in the common.

Ralph Waldo Emerson

AN IMPORTANT MESSAGE
FROM THE PUBLISHER

Each person's treatment, advice, medical aids, physical therapy and other approaches to health care are unique and highly dependant upon the diagnosis and overall assessment by the medical team.

We emphasize therefore that the information within this book is not a substitute for the advice and treatment from a health care professional.

This book provides generic information concerning the issues around confusion and common sense, well-established care practices for people who are confused.

With all this in mind, the publishers and authors disclaim any responsibility for any adverse effects resulting directly or indirectly from the suggestions contained within this book or from any misunderstanding of the content on the part of the reader.

HAVE YOU HEARD

The following are actual statements found in insurance forms where the claimants attempted to summarize the details of an accident:

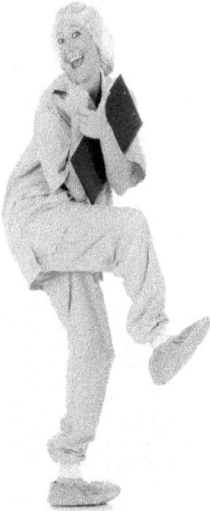

- "Coming home, I drove into the wrong house and collided with a tree I don't have."
- "The other car collided with mine without giving warning of its intention."
- "I thought my window was down, but I found out it was up when I put my head through it."
- "I collided with a stationary truck coming the other way."
- "I attempted to kill a fly, and I drove into a telephone pole."

Source: www.funnymail.com

HOW MUCH DO YOU KNOW?

It helps to figure out how much you know before you start. In this way you will have an idea as to the gaps in your knowledge prior to reading the content. Please circle to indicate the best answer. Remember, at this stage, you are not expected to know all the answers:

1. All confusion is permanent.

a. True

b. False

2. Which of the following are common causes of confusion?

a. Infections

b. Medications

c. Not enough fluids

d. All of the above

3. Which of the following symptoms are common with confusion?

a. Good attention span

b. Memory loss

c. Clear thinking

d. A and B

4. You should approach confused people from the front.

a. True

b. False

5. Which of the following would be appropriate when caring for a confused person?

a. Keep activities simple

b. Give plenty of choices

c. Set time limits for tasks

d. Keep lights off at night

6. Agitation is sometimes caused by an unmet need.

a. True

b. False

7. Confusion often improves in the evening.

a. True

b. False

ANSWERS

1. b. Confusion is often caused by a minor condition or issue.

2. d. These three factors are examples of temporary causes of confusion.

3. b. Memory loss and confusion often go hand-in-hand.

4. a. Approaching from the front does seem to help.

5. a. Simple activities reduce the chances of making the confusion worse.

6. a. Confusion can be an overreaction to an unmet need.

7. b. A confused person often becomes more confused in the evening.

WHAT IS CONFUSION?

Confusion is a common condition, particularly among older people. Confused people act in ways that can be challenging for busy caregivers. They may resist bathing, eating, and toileting. They may sleep during the day and wander during the night. They may become agitated and irritable.

Confusion is a disturbed mental state. It can last for only a short period of time or it can be permanent. There are two main types of confusion.

Delirium is confusion that lasts for a short time. It usually begins fairly quickly and ends when the cause of the confusion is removed. Although delirium often lasts less than five days, it may take several weeks for behavior to completely return to normal. Fourteen to 56% of elderly hospitalized patients experience delirium.

Dementia is confusion that lasts for a long time. It usually cannot be cured. The confusion generally worsens as time passes.

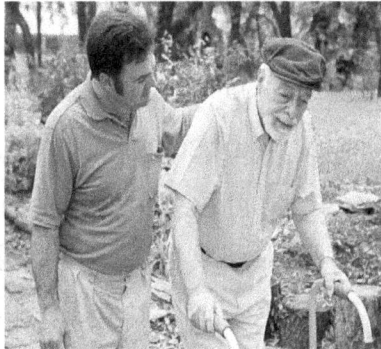

WHAT CAUSES CONFUSION?

People who are 65 years or older are more likely to develop confusion. Those who are in hospitals and those with other types of mental disorders are more at risk. Using physical restraints on people can also increase the risk of confusion.

SHORT-TERM CONFUSION

Medications are the most common cause of delirium, or short-term confusion. Some of the other possible causes of short-term confusion are:

- Infections, illnesses, and injuries
- Strange surroundings, (experienced, for example, after being admitted to a hospital)
- Loss of sleep
- Poor nutrition and not enough fluids
- Lack of stimulation, (experienced, for example, when patients are immobilized or have poor vision)
- Too much stimulation, including noisy surroundings
- Acute stress, (experienced, for example, after the loss of spouse or a change in living environment)
- A history of abuse of alcohol or drugs

Short-term confusion usually stops when the cause is removed or fixed.

LONG-TERM CONFUSION

Alzheimer's Disease is the most common cause of long-term confusion. Other possible causes include strokes and particular medical conditions.

WHAT ARE THE SYMPTOMS OF CONFUSION?

Confusion has many symptoms. Confused people have difficulty thinking clearly. Their attention span may be limited. They can be easily distracted. They have problems remembering things. Appointments and conversations are easily forgotten. People who are confused may put items in unusual places. For example, they may put the toaster in the oven or canned food in the freezer.

It may be difficult for confused people to care for themselves. They may have poor judgment. Some of their behaviors could be unsafe: wearing the wrong clothes for the weather, for example. They may stop doing regular or normal activities. Every-day tasks may become difficult. Confusion can lead to problems performing activities that involve many steps, such as cooking a meal. They may forget how to balance a checkbook.

Confused people may not know where they are. They can easily wander out of their home or health care facility and get lost. They may not be able to identify or remember where they live. They may not be able to identify the date or even the current year. For example, people may think it is 20 years earlier. They may not understand what they are seeing or hearing or they may see or hear things that are not there.

Some confused people become drowsy. They move slowly or sit and do nothing for long periods of time. They may be slow responding. Other people, however, become restless and agitated. They may repeat one movement over and over, such as banging on a table.

Emotional problems of confused people include irritability, mood swings, and being afraid and distrustful. Sleeping problems are common. Confused people often have problems communicating. They may forget simple words, use the wrong words, or not understand what is being said to them. These symptoms usually get worse during the evening or when the person is tired.

CONSIDER FOR A MOMENT . . .

Can you think of any confused people

you have known in the past?

What symptoms did they have?

SYMPTOM CHECKLIST

Difficulty thinking clearly ❏

Limited attention span ❏

Difficulty remembering things ❏

Putting items in unusual places ❏

Difficulty in caring for themselves ❏

Poor judgment ❏

Unsafe behaviour ❏

Wearing the wrong clothes ❏

Difficulty performing multi-step activities ❏

Not knowing where they are ❏

Wandering ❏

Drowsiness ❏

Moving slowly ❏

Restless/agitated ❏

Repeat the same activity ❏

Emotional problems ❏

Sleeping problems ❏

Difficulty communicating ❏

MANAGING CHALLENGING BEHAVIORS: WHAT WOULD YOU DO?

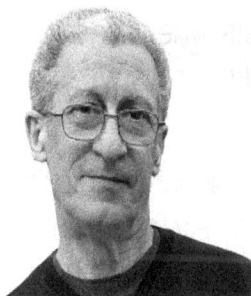

Mr. Kelly is 71 years old and has been diagnosed with Alzheimer's Disease. When Mr. Kelly could not manage on his own, he moved in with his daughter, Lynn, and her family. This living arrangement did not work out well. Lynn's father became more confused over time and his behavior became difficult to manage.

Mr. Kelly had difficulty sleeping and would wander around the house at night. His memory was poor and he would forget things. Lynn worried about this particularly because her father left the stove on several times. One night Mr. Kelly turned on the hot water tap in the kitchen and forgot to turn it off. Water flooded the kitchen floor and leaked into the rooms below.

As time passed, Lynn noticed her father become more agitated and restless. It became difficult to get him to eat. It was also hard to get him to bathe. He would yell at Lynn if she tried to convince him to do so.

Six months ago, Lynn arranged to have her father admitted to a nursing home. Since coming to the agency, Mr. Kelly's behavior has been even more difficult to manage. He often forgets where he is and what time it is. He sometimes looks for his wife who died eight years ago.

Mr. Kelly sometimes believes that he is late picking up his little girl (Lynn) from school. At those times, he becomes very upset. He has difficulty getting dressed and feeding himself. He is awake at night a lot. The staff is finding it more and more difficult to communicate with him. He wears glasses, but his hearing is good.

Which of the symptoms of confusion mentioned in the previous checklist does Mr. Kelly have?

Caring for confused people can be a challenging experience especially as they can be difficult to communicate with which adds to the problem.

What would you do if Mr. Kelly were your relative?

Everyone deserves to be treated with respect and dignity. Family and caregivers must treat Mr. Kelly with respect and dignity and be patient and flexible in trying to meet his needs.

We all value the ability to make choices in our daily lives. Mr. Kelly should be permitted to make choices whenever possible and encouraged to do as much as possible for himself.

The safety of confused clients and the staff is a big concern. It is important that Mr. Kelly be kept safe. The environment must be safe and he must be closely supervised.

Remember that short-term confusion can end if its cause is treated. Caregivers should look for possible causes of confusion. Is Mr. Kelly receiving proper nutrition and adequate fluids? Is he suffering any pain or discomfort? Is his medication producing unwanted side effects? If possible, restraints should be avoided and he should be getting enough sleep each night.

People react to their environment and the way they are treated. Mr. Kelly's environment should be caring, supportive and as calming as possible. Stress and noise should be kept to a minimum. Caregivers should always explain their activities and procedures and use routines that Mr. Kelly is familiar with. His surroundings should be as normal and as home-like as possible.

Mr. Kelly's daughter, Lynn, will also need support. She may be upset by her father's behavior. She may be feeling guilty because she cannot care for him. She should be encouraged to talk and express her feelings and she should be allowed to help with her father's care.

Sometimes, as a caregiver, you may have to get help from others. If you have questions, problems, or concerns about your family member or loved one, talk to your supervisor about him.

Let's have another look at Mr. Kelly. What specific difficulties does he have? Put yourself in the place of his caregiver and consider what you can do about the challenging behaviors on the following pages.

Communication problems

The health care staff finds it difficult to communicate with Mr. Kelly. He may use the wrong words when he is talking because he can't remember the correct ones. He may not understand what is being said to him.

Many challenging behaviors are actually attempts to communicate. Mr. Kelly may be trying to express his needs. He may be getting frustrated and agitated. Try to understand the cause of the behavior instead of trying to change the behavior. If you understand the cause of the behavior, you can then try to meet his needs.

Attempt to find out as much as you can about Mr. Kelly. What does he like to do? What are his dislikes? You will be in a better position to understand Mr. Kelly's behaviors if you know more about him.

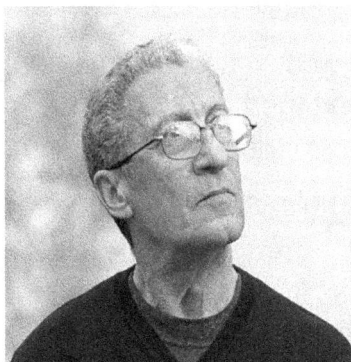

Caregivers can become frustrated trying to figure out what Mr. Kelly is trying to say. Be patient and understanding. Try these strategies when communicating with him:

- Look for non-verbal signals. What is Mr. Kelly's tone of voice? What are his facial expressions? Gestures?
- Speak slowly.
- Be calm.
- Face Mr. Kelly and maintain eye contact.
- Explain your actions.
- Use simple, familiar words.
- Use clear, short sentences.
- Allow time for Mr. Kelly to respond.
- Use nonverbal cues, such as pointing or touching. Smile.
- Repeat sentences if needed.
- Tell Mr. Kelly what you want him to do, rather than what you don't want him to do. This is often easier for the confused client to understand.
- Ask only simple questions that Mr. Kelly can answer.
- Provide only two choices or options.
- Try to keep conversation topics pleasant.

CONSIDER FOR A MOMENT . . .

Have you ever had difficulty

communication with a confused person?

Have you tried any of these strategies?

Are there other strategies you

would try next time?

Disorientation

Disorientation means not knowing where you are or what time it is. It can also mean not knowing who you are. Mr. Kelly often forgets where he is and what time it is. He looks for his deceased wife and sometimes thinks Lynn, his daughter, is still a child. This is common for confused people.

Try to orientate him to the present. Whenever you are with him, call Mr. Kelly by name. Identify the time of day by saying, "Good morning" or "Good night" and tell him what the weather is like. Encourage him to look out a window. Tell him what is happening. Talk to him about special occasions. For example, in December, talk to him about Christmas or Hanukkah.

Put a large clock and calendar in Mr. Kelly's room. A television or radio in his room will also help to keep Mr. Kelly informed about what's going on. Information boards placed around the health care unit can include the date and day of the week. Make sure Mr. Kelly wears his glasses and the lighting is good. If he needs a hearing aid, make sure he wears it and that it functions properly.

You must be careful when you are giving information to Mr. Kelly. If he does not agree with the information, he can react with anger and hostility. Don't argue with him.

Encourage Mr. Kelly's daughter and other family members to visit. Personal belongings from home may help make his room more familiar.

Difficulty sleeping

Pain, discomfort, side effects from medications, too much tea or coffee, hunger, and the need to go to the bathroom can all cause difficulty sleeping.

To promote sleep, encourage Mr. Kelly to get up at the same time every day. He should have regular activity throughout the day. Discourage afternoon napping. However, do allow Mr. Kelly to have rest periods. Make sure he doesn't get overtired.

Be careful of what Mr. Kelly eats and when he eats. Make sure he avoids sweets and caffeine during the evening. He should not eat a big meal shortly before bedtime. He may, however, sleep better with a light snack shortly before bed. Fluids should be restricted in the evening. Having to get up to go to the bathroom will interrupt his sleep.

Help Mr. Kelly establish a bedtime routine. Try to include parts of the routine he used at home. Make sure he changes into nightclothes. Make sure he uses the bathroom. A back rub or relaxation tapes may help him relax. Some people may find comfort in a stuffed animal or hearing soft music.

At night, keep lighting low. A night light may help prevent Mr. Kelly from becoming agitated if he does wake up during the night. Decrease noise, including conversation among staff. Avoid interrupting his sleep.

If Mr. Kelly does wake up agitated during the night, approach him in a calm manner. Find out if he wants anything. Remind him quietly of the time and reassure him that everything is okay.

If you suspect that Mr. Kelly's difficulty sleeping is due to pain, the medication he is taking, or a bladder condition, check with his health care professionals. If Mr. Kelly continues to stay awake at night, he may need a sleeping pill to help him relax in the evening.

CONSIDER FOR A MOMENT . . .
Does the person you're caring for
have problems sleeping?
Is there anything else you've found
that works to help them sleep?

Difficulty eating

Feeding difficulties can include forgetting to eat, forgetting how to eat, becoming distracted while eating, and having a poor appetite.

You can help Mr. Kelly by always using the same routines during mealtimes. Encourage him to sit in the same place during meals. Patterns on tablecloths and dishes can be distracting so be sure to use plain ones. Try to limit noise during mealtimes. Playing soft music, however, may help.

Find out what foods Mr. Kelly likes and dislikes. Try to include food that he likes. Limit his choices. Offer only one utensil and one dish at a time. Finger foods are good. Small, frequent meals may work better than larger meals. Provide verbal encouragement while he is eating. "That's good, Mr. Kelly. Try more of the sandwich now."

Remember safety. Ensure Mr. Kelly's food is cut into small pieces and drinks are not too hot. Remove utensils or dishes that could be dangerous. Don't rush Mr. Kelly while he is eating.

Difficulty bathing

Helping confused people meet basic needs, such as bathing, can be one of the biggest challenges. It is not uncommon for them to resist, scream, or strike out. There are a number of possible reasons for these behaviors. They may feel that bathing is unpleasant, threatening, or embarrassing. They may find the room too cold but be unable to tell you. They may be tired of waiting while you get the bath ready. Some people may be afraid of splashing water and many people resist getting their head wet.

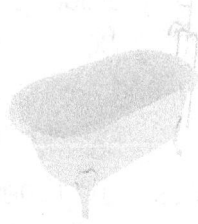

Here are some tips to help you assist Mr. Kelly bathe:

• Try to find out how Mr. Kelly normally performed this task. What did he like and dislike?

• Remain calm. Use a soft voice and smile.

• Don't scold Mr. Kelly if he argues or refuses. If he gets upset, try again later.

• Do what you can to prepare the bath before bringing Mr. Kelly into the room. Make sure towels and supplies are available. Make sure the room is warm.

- Try to let Mr. Kelly feel in control. Allow him to do whatever he can, even if it takes longer to complete the bath.

- Be flexible. Allow Mr. Kelly to make decisions if possible. Would he prefer a bath or a shower? Would he prefer a bath in the morning or evening?

- Make your requests simple. Show Mr. Kelly what you want him to do. Make the motion yourself. For example, give the washcloth to Mr. Kelly, say "Wash your face," and make the motion of washing your own face.

- Use praise when Mr. Kelly has completed a part of the task.

- Talk about pleasant topics of personal interest to Mr. Kelly. Talk about Lynn and his grandchildren.

- Avoid directing water directly onto his head. Use a hand-held shower and a gentle stream of water.

- Respect Mr. Kelly's dignity. If he is concerned about being naked, allow him to keep a towel around himself as much as possible.

- If he doesn't want a bath every day, respect his wishes. Use sponge baths between tub baths or showers.

- Be gentle. Use touch in a soothing way. Do not scrub him during the bath. Pat dry rather than rubbing.

- Remember that rushing the bath will increase Mr. Kelly's anxiety.
- Create a safe environment. Use a non-slip mat in the tub. Grab bars will help prevent falls. Make sure the water is at the right temperature. Never leave Mr. Kelly unattended in the bathtub.

Towel bath

A towel bath has also been found to be helpful for some confused people who resist personal care. The process involves placing washcloths and towels in a plastic bag and then adding warm water with no-rinse body shampoo to the bag. Using the towels and washcloths, the caregiver begins the cleansing procedure at the person's feet moving upwards. The upper body and the hands are washed last.

This bathing process provides warmth, comfort, and relaxation while cleansing in a manner that is not too invasive. If the person will tolerate the presence of two caregivers, one can talk to the person and help distract him while the other caregiver performs the bathing.

The process can be individualized to meet the needs of the individual. Keep in mind the general principles of bathing someone, such as keeping her covered as much as possible during the procedure. This may help to lessen her agitation. Other comfort measures are warm towels for drying, a heat lamp, and soft music. Try to carry out the bathing at a quiet time, with as little noise as possible in the bathing area.

Difficulty dressing and toileting

Let Mr. Kelly make some choices about what he will wear. Offer only two choices: "This shirt or that one?" Choose simple clothes that are easy to put on and take off. For example, Velcro closures are easier to use than buttons and snaps. Don't forget footwear. Make sure Mr. Kelly is wearing footwear that is safe and appropriate.

Lay out the clothes that Mr. Kelly will be wearing on his bed. If needed, assist him by passing the clothes to him item by item. Let Mr. Kelly do as much as possible on his own. Don't rush him. You may need to post signs or posters in his room showing how to put certain items on. Or you can post signs that outline the order that clothes should be put on.

Toileting can be a common problem for many confused people. They may forget where the bathroom is. They may not be able to get their clothes off. Some medications and some medical conditions can lead to the need to get to the bathroom quickly which can lead to accidents. If Mr. Kelly does have an accident, treat him with dignity and respect. Do not embarrass him. Reassure him that you do not mind helping him.

Make sure he goes to the bathroom on a regular basis. Watch for signs that he needs to go to the bathroom — restlessness, for example. Encourage him to wear clothes he can remove quickly. Limit the amount of fluids he drinks in the evening. Put signs and pictures on the bathroom door to show him where the bathroom is.

Agitation, restlessness, and wandering

Mr. Kelly is becoming more and more agitated and restless. Agitation and restlessness are often the result of an unmet need or of feelings of anxiety. Fear, pain, discomfort, or certain medications can cause agitation. Having too much going on around them can lead to agitation. Not fully understanding what is going on—because of poor vision or difficulty hearing—can also lead to agitation. People who are agitated are often restless. They may repeat certain actions, such as banging the arm of a chair.

Try to determine why Mr. Kelly is agitated. Is he hungry, cold, afraid, or tired? Try to reduce Mr. Kelly's stress. Reduce noise and distractions. Use routines that are familiar to him as much as possible. Avoid moving Mr. Kelly to unfamiliar environments. Ensure he wears his glasses. Provide rest periods during the day.

Approach Mr. Kelly from the front if he is agitated. Use touch. Keep calm. Maintain eye contact. Try to distract Mr. Kelly when he gets agitated. Give him a simple task to do, such as folding clothes or watering plants. Soothing music may help.

Reminiscence, remembering one's past, is a common activity, especially among older people. Memories reinforce our sense of who we are. They can be shared with others. For some people, memories can provide a sense of comfort and can reduce restlessness and agitation. On the other hand, some people do not want to remember the past because of painful memories. Knowing about Mr. Kelly's past may help you understand his behavior.

Confused people often wander, especially if they are agitated or restless. If Mr. Kelly begins to wander, encourage regular exercise and activity. Reassure him that he is okay and in the right place. Distract him by suggesting another activity or by offering a snack.

Maintain a safe environment. Supervise him closely. Keep exterior doors locked. Alarms should be installed on doors.

If a family member who wanders lives at home, neighbors should have contact names and numbers in case they see her wandering outside. Ensure that she wears a Medic Alert bracelet with her name, address, and telephone number on it. Dangerous tools and matches should be kept out of her reach.

CONSIDER FOR A MOMENT . . .

If your loved one lives in a

health care facility, does the facility

have policies about how to

deal with wandering behaviors,

including what to do if a

client goes missing?

If so, what do these policies say?

Aggressiveness and hostility

Mr. Kelly is not showing any signs of physical aggression. However, he has been hostile and verbally aggressive.

Try to find out why Mr. Kelly is showing signs of aggression. Fear can cause verbal and physical aggressiveness. Is he afraid of something? Reduce noise and activity around Mr. Kelly. Keep your requests simple. Try to use the same routines with him. Explain your activities and procedures. Try to make him as comfortable as possible.

When faced with physical or verbal aggression, use clear communication. Do not argue with Mr. Kelly. Reassure him that he is safe. Move slowly and encourage talk rather than action. Try to calmly remove Mr. Kelly from the situation. Try distracting him. Take him for a walk or out to get a snack. Confused people are usually easy to distract. If you think Mr. Kelly's behavior could become violent, take measures to ensure his safety and the safety of others. If necessary, notify other staff members or call for help.

CONSIDER FOR A MOMENT . . .
If your family member lives in
a health care facility, does
the facility have a policy on
the management of aggressive
behaviour by confused clients?
If so, what does it say?

Storing objects

Some confused people store small objects such as pens, coins, or socks. If Mr. Kelly is doing this, try to find out where he is putting the items. He may be using pockets, drawers, or shoes. If the behavior doesn't cause a problem, don't worry about it. It may be a source of comfort to him. However, Mr. Kelly may get attached to a dangerous object, such as a knife. If so, replace it with something safe. Lock up dangerous or valuable items. Remove items that can cause a problem if hoarded, such as food that will spoil.

CONSIDER FOR A MOMENT . . .

Have you ever cared for a person
who stored items?
What items did he or she
store and where?
What did you do about it?
How did the person react?

Sundowning

Sundowning is a term for increased confusion in the late afternoon and evening. Lack of stimulation is a common cause. It can also happen when the person is overtired.

To prevent sundowning, ensure that Mr. Kelly has rest periods throughout the day. Encourage him to wear his glasses. Make sure the lighting in his room is neither too bright nor too dim.

Make sure that Mr. Kelly gets some stimulation. For example, leave the radio on in his room during the day. Be careful, though, that he does not get too much stimulation.

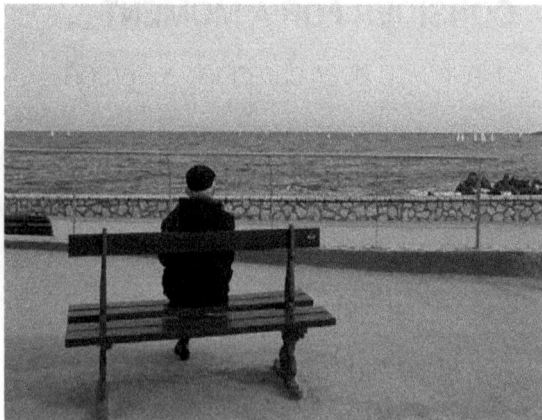

10 tips for communicating with confused people

1. Look at non-verbal signals, such as tone of voice, facial expression, and gestures, to try and understand what the person wants to say.

2. Calmly face the person and maintain eye contact.

3. Use simple and familiar words to explain what you are about to do. Repeat sentences if needed.

4. Use clear, short sentences and speak slowly.

5. Try not to rush. Allow the person time to respond.

6. Use nonverbal cues, such as pointing or touching, to help the person understand what you are saying.

7. Say what you want the person to do, rather than what you don't want her to do. This is often easier for confused people to understand.

8. If you need to ask questions, keep them simple.

9. Provide only 2 choices or options.

10. Support the person's attempts to communicate. Try to keep conversation topics pleasant. Remember to smile!

CASE EXAMPLE

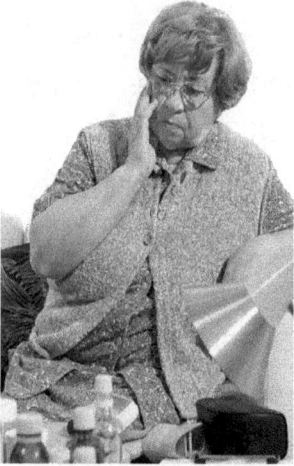

Mrs. Burry is 75 years old. She lives alone in her own home. Usually, she cares for herself quite well. For the past several weeks, however, she has had a severe chest infection. She refuses to go to hospital. She is, however, taking medications ordered by her doctor.

Her family has noticed that Mrs. Burry has not been able to care for herself while she has been sick. She spends a lot of time in bed or sitting in a chair in the living room. They don't think she is bathing or changing her clothes. They also noticed that she is sometimes confused. She is forgetting things. She is also mixing up the time and day of the week. Last week a neighbor called Mrs. Burry's daughter. Mrs. Burry was wandering down the street wearing only a thin nightgown and slippers. That's when her family called the home care agency for help.

Imagine that you are Mrs. Burry's caregiver. What should you do?

YOUR ANSWERS TO CASE EXAMPLE

SUGGESTED ANSWERS TO CASE EXAMPLE

You should realize that Mrs. Burry's confusion is probably related to her infection. The medications she's now taking may also cause confusion. She may be eating and drinking poorly. She may not be sleeping. She may be having some pain. You should monitor her nutrition, the amount of fluids she drinks, and her sleeping. Ask her if she is having pain.

Treat Mrs. Burry with respect and dignity. Communicate clearly. Ensure her needs are being met. Assist her with eating, bathing, changing her clothes, and toileting. Be calm, patient, and flexible as you help her. Try to find out her normal routines from her family. Follow these familiar routines. Allow her to make decisions and to do as much as she can.

Look for possible safety problems in her environment. Ensure the lighting is good. Supervise her closely. Try to distract her if she starts to wander. Look for things that could cause her to fall. What kinds of locks are on the doors? Does she walk directly onto the street or into a fenced yard? Talk to her family if there is anything in her house that you think is not safe.

If you think the medications could be increasing the confusion, talk to the health care professional. As well, mention your concern for Mrs. Burry's safety.

CONCLUSION

Confusion is a common condition among elderly people whether they are cared for in nursing homes, hospitals, or their own homes. Frequently, these confused people may have challenging behaviors.

The goal for the caregiver is to meet that person's needs. As we have seen, there are many strategies to help you manage challenging behaviors. Try to find out the cause of challenging behaviors. Keep the environment safe. Supervise confused people closely. Treat them with dignity and respect. Good communication is important. Remain calm, patient, and flexible.

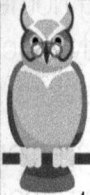

CHECK YOUR KNOWLEDGE

1. Define confusion, reminiscence, and sundowning.

2. Identify four causes of confusion.

3. Identify four symptoms that are common in confused people.

4. Describe three strategies to help orient a confused person.

5. How can you improve communication with a confused person?

6. Discuss five strategies for assisting a confused person with a bath.

7. What should you do if a confused person becomes agitated?

TEST YOURSELF

Please circle to indicate the best answer:

1. Elderly people are more likely to get confused.
a. True
b. False

2. Medications are the most common reversible cause of confusion.
a. True
b. False

3. What can contribute to eating problems in confused people?
a. A well-lit room.
b. Lots of activity in the dining room.
c. Providing only a few choices at mealtime.
d. Providing finger food.

4. Which of the following strategies would help the people to sleep?

a. Encourage exercise during the day.

b. Avoid all bedtime snacks.

c. Vary bedtime schedule.

d. A and C.

5. You should use simple explanations and requests with confused people.

a. True

b. False

6. Keeping all the lights off at night is a good strategy when caring for confused people.

a. True

b. False

7. It is difficult to distract a confused, agitated person.

a. True

b. False

ANSWERS

1. a.True. Confusion is a common condition among elderly people who are cared for in nursing homes, hospitals, or their own homes.

2. a.True. Medications are the most common cause of delirium, or short-term confusion. The confusion usually stops when the cause is removed or fixed.

3. b.Try to limit noise and other distractions during mealtimes. Having too much going on around them can lead to agitation.

4. a.If possible, people should have regular activity throughout the day.

5. a.True. Keep your requests simple. Try to use the same routines with the person in your care and explain your activities and procedures.

6. b.False. A night light may help prevent a person from becoming agitated if she wakes up during the night.

7. b.False. The attention span of confused people may be limited; they can be easily distracted.

REFERENCES

Alzheimer's Association. (2000). Diagnostic procedures. Retrieved August 28, 2001 from http://www.alz.org/hc/diagnosing/procedures.htm

(2001). Ten warning signs. Retrieved August 28, 2001 from http://www.alz.org/caregiver/understanding/10warnings.htm

ALZwell. (1995-2001). Ways of managing severe confusion behaviors. Excerpt from C. Rob, The caregiver's guide: Helping elderly relatives cope with health and safety problems. Retrieved July 23, 2001 from http://www.webcom.com/susan/cguide.html

Encyclopedia of the Self. (1999-2001). Dictionary information – Definition confusion. Retrieved July 23, 2001 from http://www.selfknowledge.com/109729.htm

Espino, D.V., Jules-Bradley, A.C., Johnston, C.L, & Mouton, C.P. (1998). Diagnostic approach to the confused elderly patient. American Family Practice, 57(6).

Foreman, M.D., Mion, L.C., Tryostad, L., Fletcher, K., & the NICHE Faculty. (1999). Standard of practice protocol: Acute confusion/delirium. Geriatric Nursing, 20(3).

Ludwick, R. (1999). Clinical decision making: Recognition of confusion and application of restraints. Orthopaedic Nursing, 18(1).

Malik, N. (2000, May). Delirium, sign of an underlying life-threatening condition. Geriatrics & Aging, 3(4). Retrieved August 24, 2001 from http://www.geriatricsandaging.ca

McDonald, M. (1999). Assessment and management of cancer pain in the cognitively impaired elderly. Geriatric Nurse, 20(5).

Parke, B. (2000). Managing older confused hospital patients. Nursing BC, 32(2).

Roberts, B.L. (2001). Managing delirium in adult intensive care patients. Critical Care Nurse, 21(1).

Woodrow, P. (1998). Interventions for confusion and dementia 1: quality of life. British Journal of Nursing, 7(15).World Health Organization. (1999). Preventing acute confusion in the elderly. Bulletin of the World Health Organization. Retrieved July 23, 2001 from http://who.int/bulletin/news/vol.77no.5/confusion.html

www.ingramcontent.com/pod-product-compliance
Lightning Source LLC
Chambersburg PA
CBHW060646280326
41933CB00012B/2176